What Makes Me
Happy, Healthy, and Alive?

Teresa Wolfe
Illustrations by Marcia Fajardo

outskirts
press

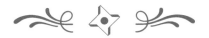

This Book Belongs to:

_____

What makes me healthy, happy and alive?

I need ...

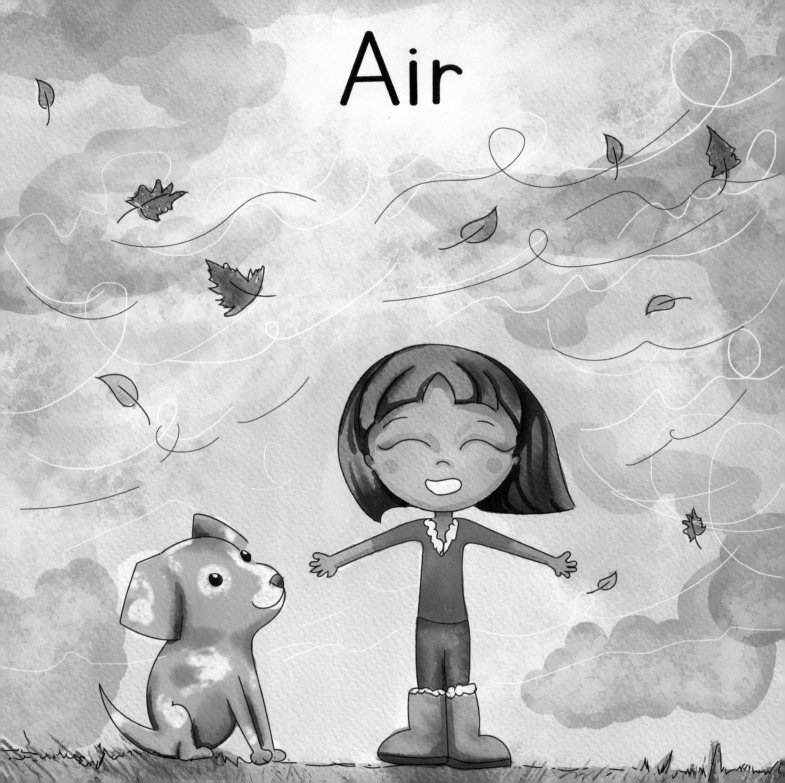

I need ...

Water

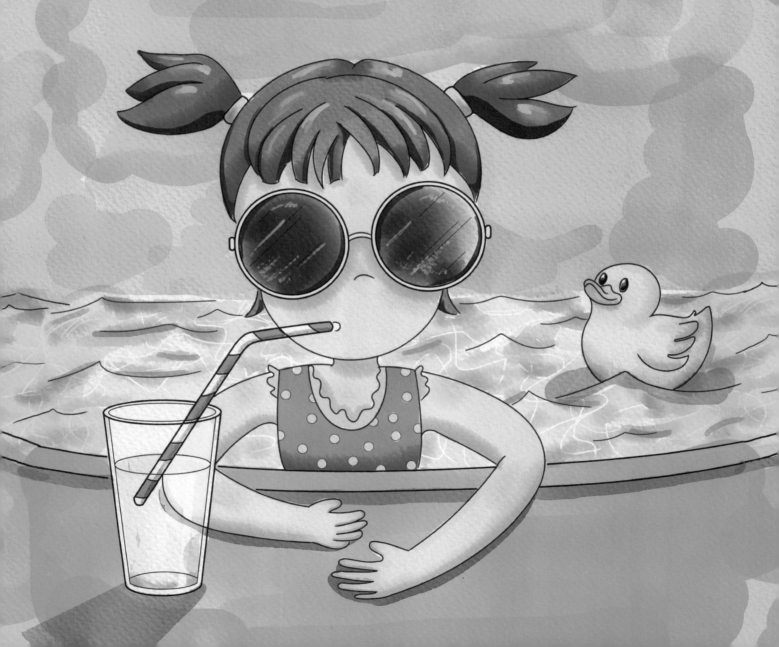

I need ...

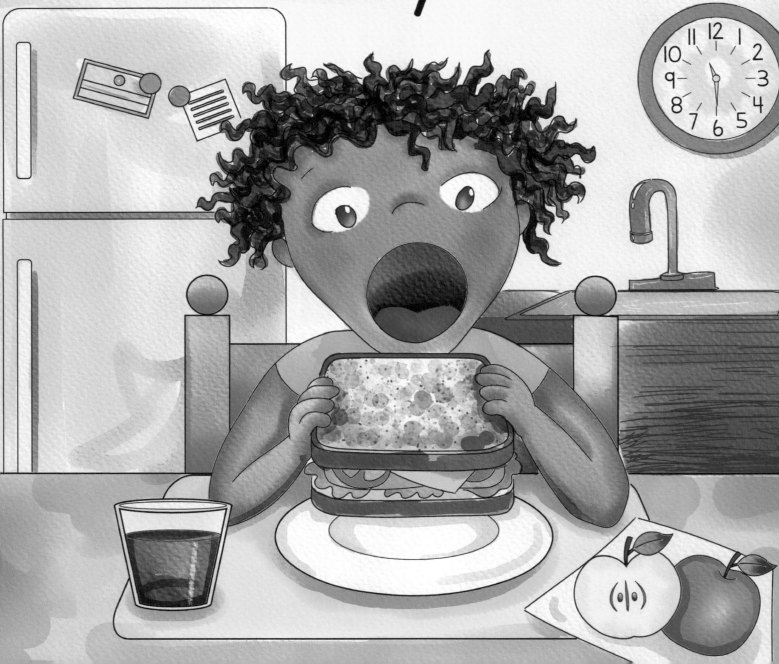

I need ...

Rest

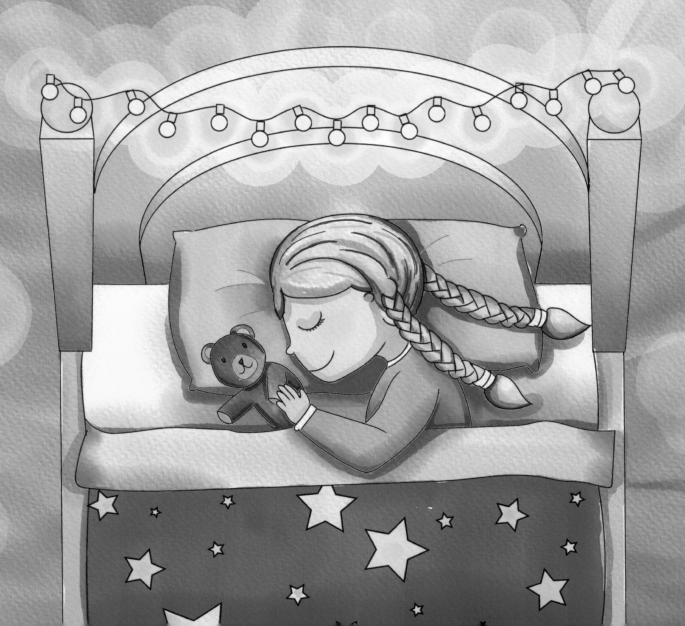

I need ...

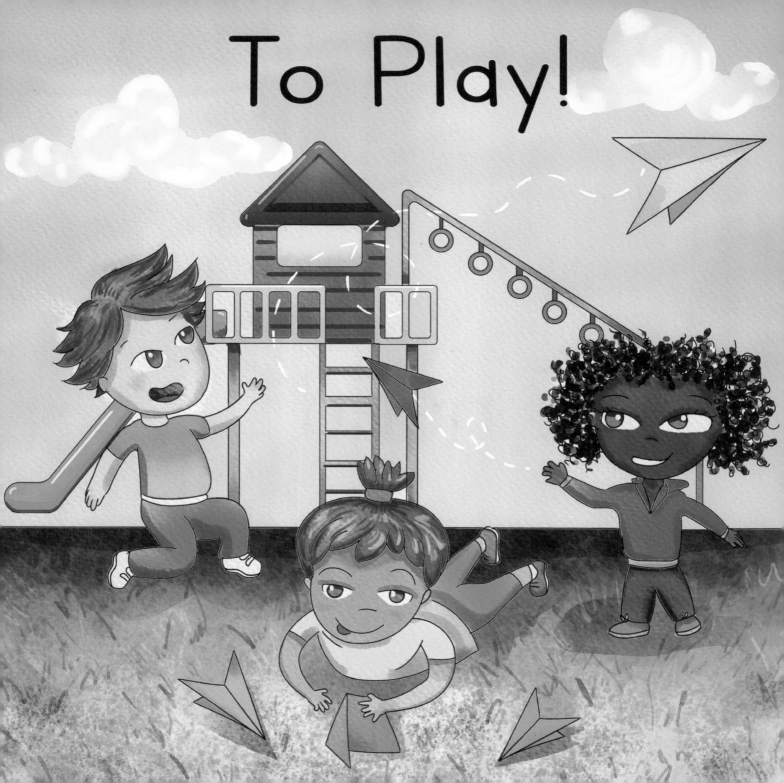

I need ...

Family

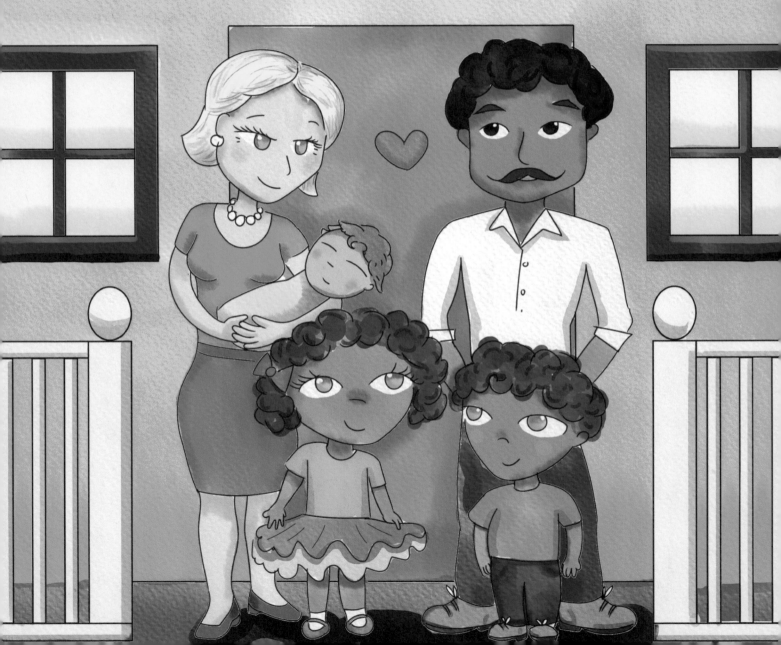

I need ...

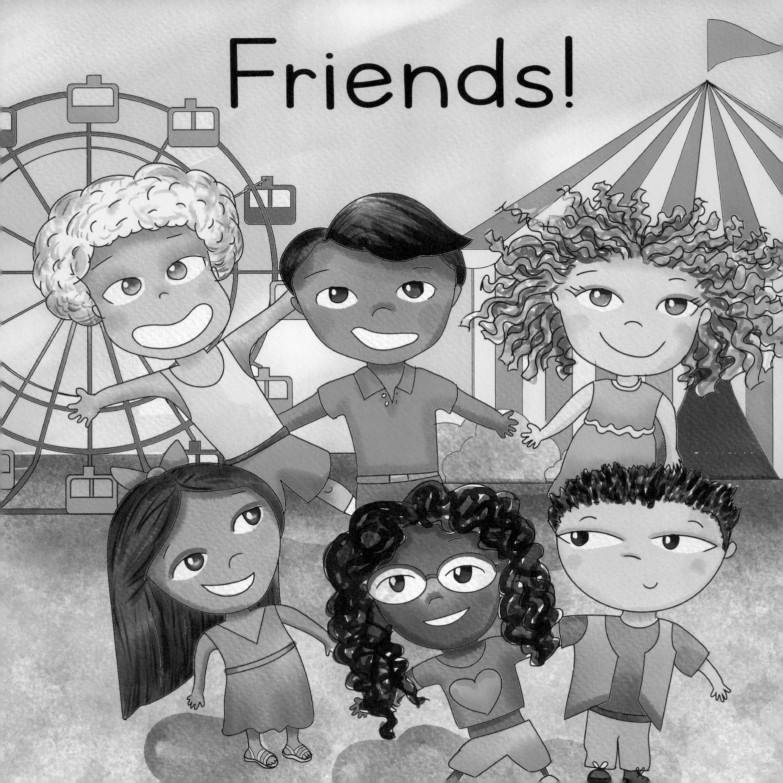

I need ...

Exercise

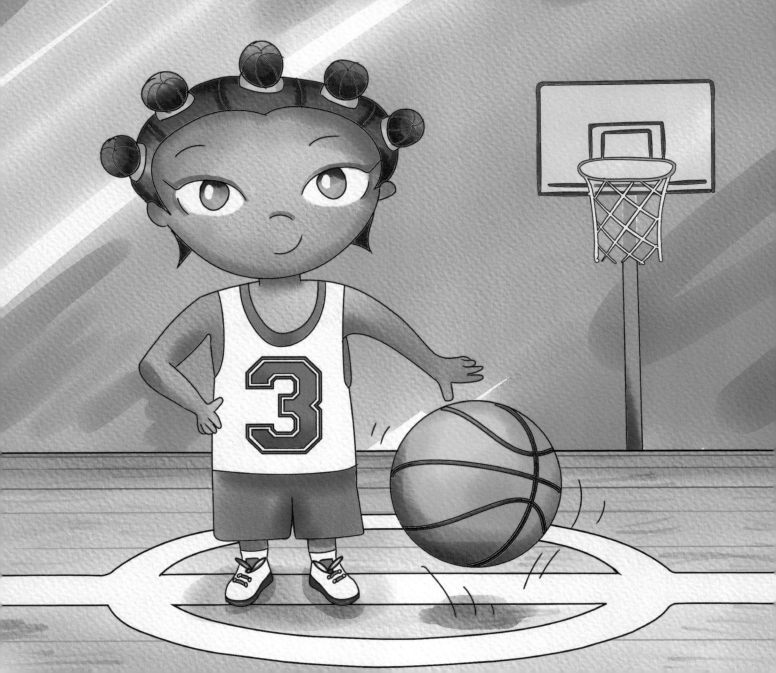

I need ...

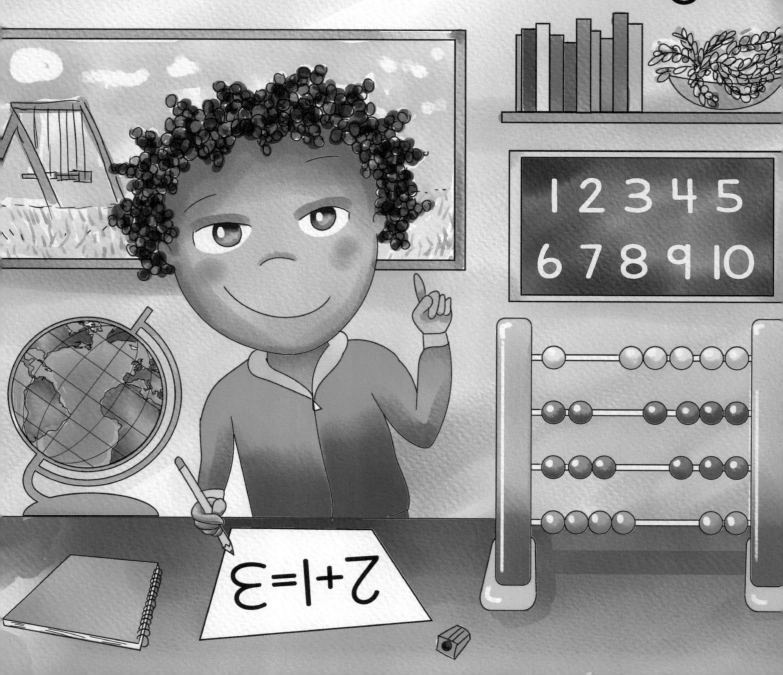

I need ...

To Create

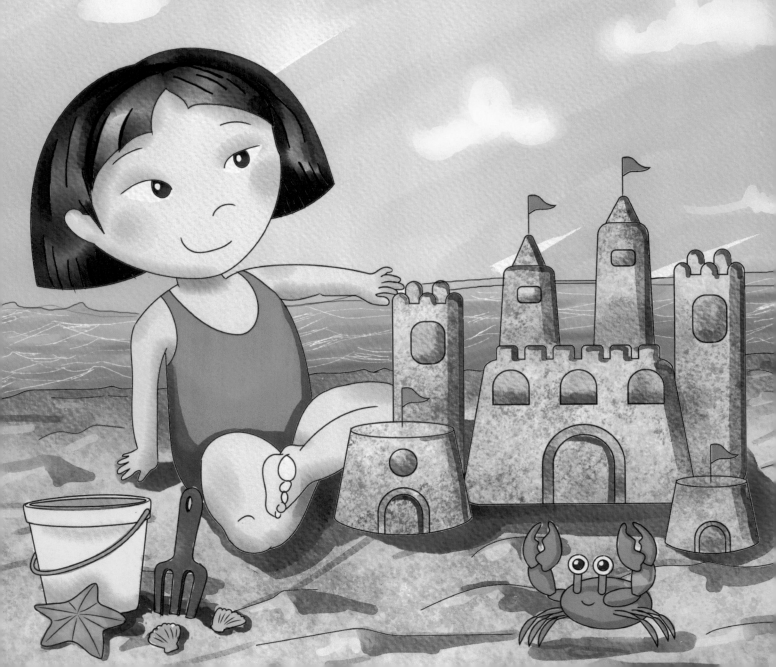

I need ...

To Feel Helpful

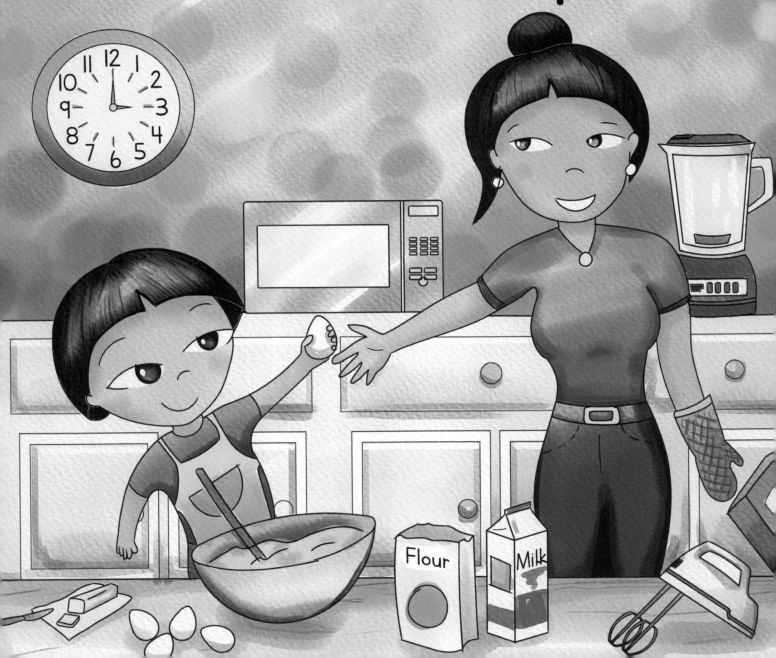

I need ...

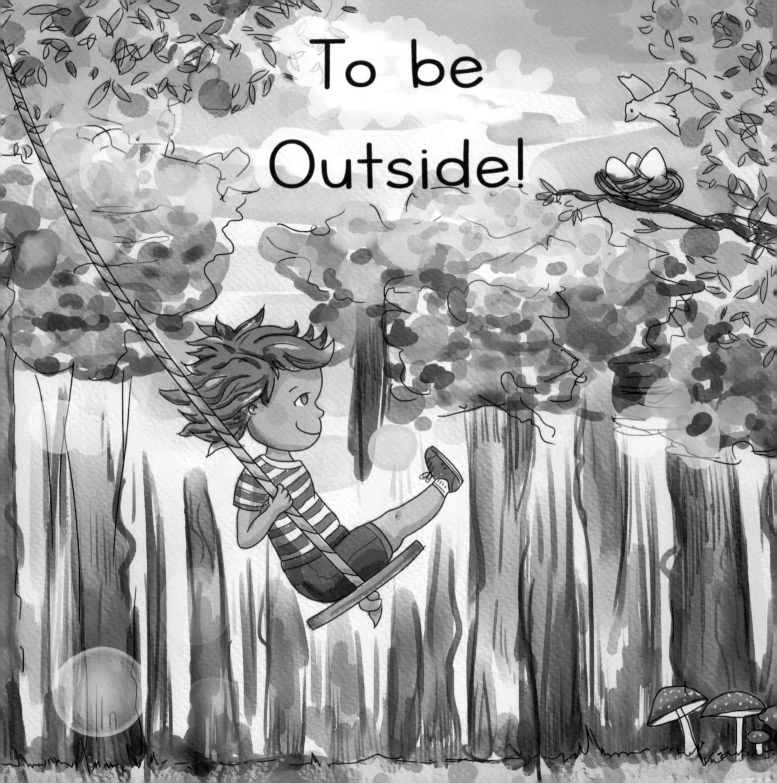

To be
Outside!

I need ...

My Special Things

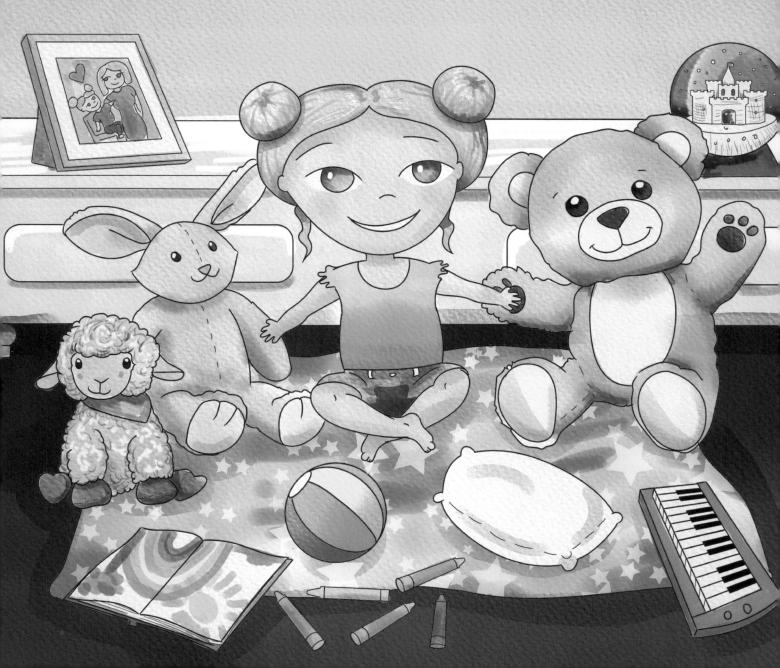

I need ...

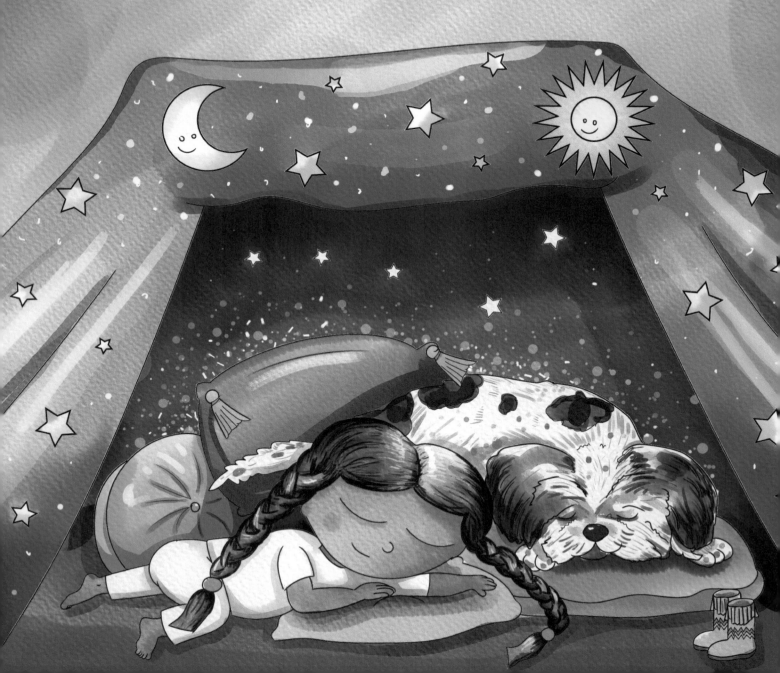

To Feel Safe

But most of all, I need and want to give ...

Love

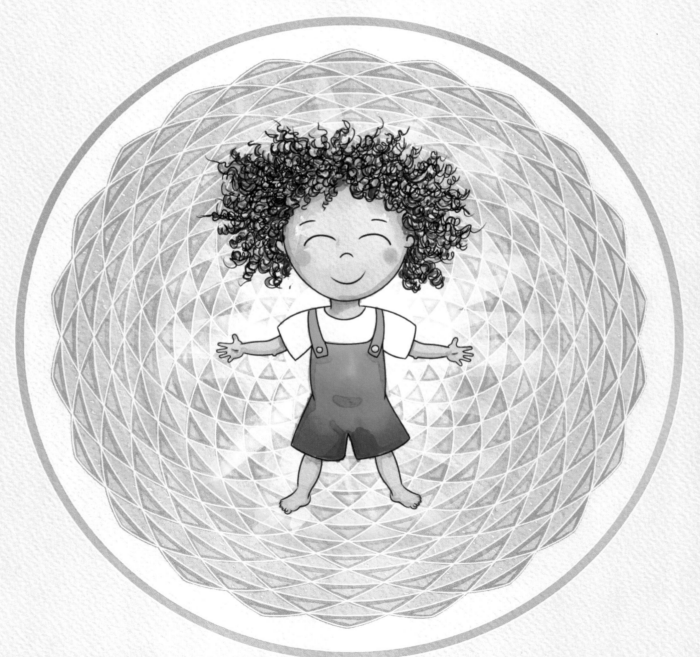

What Makes Me Happy, Healthy, and Alive?

Author Interview

1. What inspired you to write this book?

My deepest passion is to be an ambassador of goodwill and promote individual and environmental health on a global scale. As a food scientist and eco-herbalist, I have presented hundreds of programs over the years on health and well-being with a focus on good nutrition. This concept has evolved over time from underscoring the need for good nutrition to promoting nourishment. They are not the same.

In 2016, I presented a program (one for adults and another for children) titled "Genuinely Fed, on an Inner and Outer Level" at my church. The program explored the notion that healthy food is not all we need to thrive and posed questions beyond the usual scope of nutrition. I asked the adults the following questions:

What does it mean to be "nourished"?

What are the ways in which we nourish ourselves?

If we nourish ourselves at the expense of others and/or the land, are we genuinely nourished?

How can we nourish ourselves and all beings on the planet?

Can we do so sustainably?

The answers to these questions often lead people to understand what it is they need to thrive in this world. To truly thrive and be nourished, we need love, family, community, and financial resources. Beyond safety and survival, we require spiritual nourishment as well as opportunities to grow, create, contribute, and have fun.

For the children's portion of the program, I created *What Makes Me Happy, Healthy, and Alive?* as a companion to the presentation. The kids responded well to the book, enthusiastically commenting about how the concepts related to their lives as I read it to them. Parents and grandparents liked it so much that some of them took it to local schools and read it to the young children they were tutoring. Many suggested that I publish it. And so here we are.

For the published version, I have collaborated with Marcia Fajardo, a wonderful artist from Mexico City. The words of the book are deliberately simple. The illustrations are what give it substance and life. She did a fantastic job! I deeply appreciate the depth of thought, feeling, and intent she put into her work. For instance, in the illustration for feeling safe, she did not show anyone holding or comforting the child as you might expect. Sadly, not all children receive this kind of attention. Marcia and I wanted to visually suggest that children are capable of creating a safe place for themselves.

My favorite of illustration of all is the one for love. Here is how she described it: "This one (illustration) is for Love. I wanted to portray an image where kids are self-reliable and free to love regardless of the object of their attention and show how their source of love is within themselves."

2. How did you get from Teresa Wolfe, food scientist, to Teresa Wolfe, author of a book for children?

After earning my bachelor's degree, I was accepted into a doctorate program for microbiology at University of California–Berkeley. It was one of the top two microbiology programs in the country at the time and quite an honor to get in. But my financial situation dictated that I work for a while instead. I landed a job in Minneapolis at Peavey Company Flour Mills (a Fortune 500 company) as the quality control microbiologist and, later, in chemical analysis. While with Peavey, I earned a master's degree in food science and nutrition at the University of Minnesota–St. Paul. My thesis research involved studying the genetics behind the bacteria used in making fermented dairy products. What more could I want? I got to play scientist, do something practical (in the field of nutrition), and apply the skills I had learned in college. Yet, somewhere deep within, I was discontent.

After graduate school, I was hired as a faculty member for the University of Minnesota doing full-time research in the then-new field of genetic engineering. The job was ideal for my left-brained, scientific nature.

I had status and was making a good salary. Despite this, the discontent within me grew. This was not my calling.

About this time, my interest pivoted from making processed foods as a food scientist to experimenting with whole, organically grown foods. I used my training as a food scientist to invent recipes that substituted wholesome ingredients for the sugar-laden, nutrient-poor foods I had grown up eating—and that had virtually ruined my digestive tract by age twenty-two. In so doing—and to my utter delight—my personal health improved.

When I became pregnant with my first child, I left my position with the University of Minnesota. I did not feel it was good to expose a growing fetus to the chemicals, carcinogens, and radiation that were customary protocol for the research I was doing. I happened upon a job at a nature center—a total switch of gears! I thoroughly enjoyed being out of doors, and my practical side thrived on educating people regarding natural history, ecology, conservation, and the importance of a planetwide-balanced ecosystem. I viscerally integrated being connected with nature and eating wholesome foods. I became intrigued with using wild plants, first as food and then as medicine. I took up the study of herbalism.

I studied with a passion. Using my training as a scientist to set up experiments, I dutifully recorded everything. I assembled a science laboratory in my house and developed an entire line of original herbal formulas. Whenever someone in the house was ill or injured, I just went into the "herb shop" and made up some concoction that would ease their discomfort and promote healing. Our entire family medicine chest consisted of my formulas, and eventually I went into business marketing them.

In 2005, I took a part-time job with the National Park Service (NPS), hoping to learn more about the plants in the area, which would enhance my expertise as an eco-herbalist. I was so delighted and uplifted to discover the deep passion my coworkers shared for environmental preservation that I stayed with the NPS for more than nine years—initially in education and interpretation and then in resource management.

My passion to promote the health and well-being of humanity and the planet continued to grow. In 2015, I launched Global Healing Project 1, an annual Earth Day event in which everyone everywhere is asked to take *one minute* to go within and be inspired to do *one thing*, *one time* to make the world a better place. The idea is to create a critical mass of a single intent: restoration of health and balance to the Earth. To learn more, visit TeresaWolfe.com/project-1/.

This takes you up to March 13, 2016, the day I made the presentation that included a rougher version of this book in hopes that it, too, would contribute to making the world a better place. All the discontent and career switches have woven into the tapestry that I now am. The many twists and turns have given me a unique perspective on the need to nourish humanity *and the environment*. My life experience has led me to the firm belief that "A happy *you* equals a happy planet."

3.   Why do you call yourself an "eco-herbalist"?

This is a title I gave myself. It reflects my commitment to keep my herbal practices sustainable and Earth friendly. I will not use rare or endangered species or plants that have been treated with pesticides in my products.

4.   What do you hope children will take away from this book?

My takeaway message for children (and everyone) is an awareness of the basic elements needed for a wholesome life. My desire is for children to get an ingrained notion of the basic needs that must be met if they are to thrive and be happy—and that it is okay to expect these needs to be met. I want all parents and caregivers to have this same awareness and to realize it is their responsibility to fill these basic needs for their children.

I want children as young as toddlers to be exposed to and embrace these ideas so that as they go through life, they will know how important it is to fulfill their needs. Someday, they may become parents or caregivers and can continue the cycle. Every child deserves to understand the message presented in *What Makes Me Healthy, Happy, and Alive?*—for their own sake as well as the planet's.

CPSIA information can be obtained
at www.ICGtesting.com
Printed in the USA
BVHW021727260321
603114BV00002B/5